HABIT HEROES

HABIT HEROES

Building the Life You Want One Habit at a Time

T.J. RAVENSCROFT

QuillQuest Publishers

CONTENTS

1	Introduction	1
2	Understanding Habits	3
3	Identifying Your Habits	7
4	Creating Positive Habits	11
5	Breaking Negative Habits	15
6	Habit Stacking and Habit Tracking	20
7	The Power of Habit in Personal Development	24
8	Habit Heroes: Real Life Success Stories	28

Copyright © 2024 by T.J. Ravenscroft

All rights reserved. No part of this book may be reproduced in any manner whatsoever without written permission except in the case of brief quotations embodied in critical articles and reviews.

First Printing, 2024

CHAPTER 1

Introduction

The same process underlies the habitual acts, thoughts, and feelings that help or hinder your ability to thrive and meet peak potential in any and every endeavor. Humans store partial lessons, such as how to deal with feelings of happiness, sadness, anger, or anxiety, on how to entertain oneself, make initial judgments about others, and effectively save energy. The process is an incredibly automatic action-thought-emotion loop built of a series of refined "chunks" of strong synaptic connections to each other. Some of these strong connections are internally motivated, meaning that the person does it for themselves, or some are externally motivated, meaning that the person did it because they thought it was likely to improve a situation. It is the completed action-thought-emotion response that makes an experience a learning event worthy of being integrated into the action-thought-emotion loops that guide what happens to change behavior. Each learning experience eventually strengthens the neural connections involved in that experience, strengthening these connections and fine-tuning the current action, thought, and emotions in the person's environment. Other factors such as meeting basic survival and safety needs, the organization of meaningful experiences, and the repetition of behaviors being set to the rhythms of structured schedules during the lifespan also facilitate connections in Act-Think-Feel loops.

Underneath all human brain activity is the basis of survival, specifically looking good, feeling good, and being with the in-crowd to help you stay alive and thrive. Your brain has numerous ways to make sure that you continue to think and behave in routine ways, spotting familiar actions and thoughts as quickly as possible, so that effort does not have to be spent on reflexive survival responses. This is how you are able to drive to a familiar location and not remember parts of the trip. The brain underlies this amazing dynamic process by continually scanning saved visual data, unconscious preferences, heuristics, stereotypes, or rules of thumb to guide your attention and actions.

The wonderful news about your brain is that your thoughts, emotions, and actions perform together in a chemical symphony. One thought can set off waves of neurons that fire in sequences, releasing chemicals that can make you think, feel, act, and think again in about 30 seconds. Repeating this chemical dance can reinforce habituated thinking patterns to the point that action, thought, and feelings happen before you are aware of doing them.

CHAPTER 2

Understanding Habits

These all happen because of a hint that made someone know what to do without even thinking about it. These habits were ingrained into your lifestyle because the brain's habit system never goes quiet. It is always tracking the cycle of cues, routines, and rewards. And it's always trying to create and change habits. That's why your habit will always come back even if it is something you never wanted. To really understand our habits, we have to also understand the cues and the rewards that play such a big role in these cycles. And that's where a friend with a cigarette and chocolate muffins triggers our need for a smoke and sweets. They have a habit when they are forced with the soya blue cheese salad every time they order lunch and finish their meal with a chocolate sundae that contains the same amount of calories. When they're just eating a sundae or the dessert that's a reminder, it indicates a green light to order office dessert. When you are forced with a choice of double fudge bunt cake and fruit, you will leave the strawberry cake and you're going to leave dessert.

When you lose your keys, you might be out of time and your cortisol shoots up, and you use a completely different part of your brain that goes into overdrive: the prefrontal cortex. And when it does, you forget where your keys are. But when you have a habit like brushing your teeth in the morning, the basal ganglia run that automatically and perform that same behavior every time. The prefrontal cortex also helps with learning new habits by making decisions and thinking about the future. And that's a good thing if you're going to beat your habits and not reinforce the bad ones. So why is it so hard to beat our habits? Every time a habit occurs, the basal ganglia and the prefrontal cortex work together to strengthen the habit loop. A hint sparks the part of our brain to get ready for the behavior and increases the chance that the behavior will follow. Think about biting your nails, lighting a cigarette, or eating chips while watching TV.

2.1. What are habits?

There are different habits based on a person's thinking and the cultures that they bear. People always want to follow the habits that they prefer and will show much interest in the ones they have already been following. Every person's character is built by the previous habits that they used to follow from their generations. This is the reason why people show more interest in following a cultural habit of their own. Every person's habits merely depend on the culture they are following. People show more interest towards cultural activities and love to follow them. We cannot make a change if we are true lovers of our culture. But still, often we see several people in discussion trying to make some changes to their habits.

A habit is a repetitive practice or concept that most of us have when we do things. Habits have an immense power that can change our world from good to bad or from bad to good in a gradual manner, the way we practice them. Our habits differ in nature; people have both positive and negative habits. Some want to get out of them, but most of us find difficulties in replacing them. Habits are made to show what's in us and create a label in society and among ourselves. Often, the words "habits" and "cultures" are inter-related. Habits are one's preference to follow a concept, person, or thing that they are interested in. So, what are the different habits?

2.2. How habits are formed

The only reliable consensus showed in the reviewed studies was that how long it takes varies depending on the desired habits. Normalizing a new behavior into your everyday habits can take anywhere between 18 days and a whole year. You are more likely to turn the desired behavior into a habit if it is something you perform frequently. For example, it will be easier for you to start eating fruits every day than it would be to start going for a two-mile run every day if you are a couch potato. In order to form a habit, you usually have to repeat the action every day for at least 66 days in a row, but on average it takes about 90 days. After the habit has formed, you still have to perform the behavior at a constant pace, or it will in time die out. You may not notice your daily junk mail in your mailbox until you start clearing it every afternoon. Gradually the way you interact with your mail changes and you start cleaning the mailbox every day when you arrive home.

How you form habits is a bit hazy. When asked how long it takes before a specific action becomes a habit, people usually answer with a specific amount of time that you have to repeat the action before it becomes automatic: 21 days, 30 days or the seemingly most common answer, "it depends". This belief of a specific time frame being essential for something to turn into a habit has a foundation much firmer than in scientific consensus. In 2009, researchers at the University of Southern California and the Australian National University reviewed 96 studies on how long it takes to form a habit.

2.3. The power of habits

In addition to leading to success, habits also distinguish formations of strong moral character from weak character. Marcus Antonius, the Roman orator and second triumvir in Ancient Rome, told the crowds in the Athenian marketplace, "We become just by doing just acts, temperate by doing temperate acts, brave by doing brave acts." Aristotle expressed a similar sentiment: "We are what we repeatedly do. Excellence, then, is not an act, but a habit." The activities of the successful people we have mentioned earlier are borne out of strong moral character. Aristotle would not disagree with the speculation that the path to forming the habits that lead to success and happiness may be, as Thomas Aquinas (1224/5–1274) hinted, "a planted with what is morally good, being tended with good care, and a watered with the tears of repentance."

While habits can sometimes be frustrating or limiting, the idea that once a habit is formed, it can become second nature is incredibly powerful. Indeed, the significance of habits in the lives of successful people is clearly recognized. The late U.S. Senator Paul Tsongas declared, "Quality is not an act, it is a habit." Jim Ryun, the world record holder in the mile when he was only nineteen years old, wrote, "Motivation is what gets you started. Habit is what keeps you going." Similarly, Henry van Dyke, an American clergyman and writer, is often credited with suggesting, "Regularity in the hours of rising and retiring, perseverance in exercise, adaptation of dress to the variations of climate, simple and nutritious diet, and attention to the preservation of the general health, will be found, when the soul is free, or that constitution is most capable of leisure, to be sources of literary, scientific, or artistic achievements" [emphasis added].

CHAPTER 3

Identifying Your Habits

During the previous chapter, definitions for the terms habit, habit formation, behavior change, and identity-based habit formation were provided. The definitions outlined were put in place in order to examine their properties and then reveal more about their nature. Once these ideas are contemplated in depth, the analysis will be used to develop a detailed plan on how you can positively and personally change your behavior. Behavior change will then lead to a new representation of the self and as a result, create transformation of your social sphere. The idea of transformation is then used as the center point. If the definitions and subsequent processes are carried out in a method that is consistent with the transformation process, development should happen with ease. As it is with changes in behavior, significant changes in beliefs and values form the basis for the long term ability to support a new or more constructive person.

1. Does this habit pull me somewhere I want to go or is it continually pushing me away from my desired destination? Do not consider the behavior of the person who exhibits the habit. Only pay attention to whether or not the habit is aligned

with your own personal goals. 2. Who will I become because of this habit? Will I feel proud of where I have been led as a result of this repeated behavior? 3. Is this a manageable habit or habit goal? The manageable habit falls in line with the idea of baby steps. A manageable habit goal is the equivalent of taking this habit on a test drive, or an arrival fall of this habit. Once you can answer these three questions you will be able to close the gap between whom you are and who you want to become, simultaneously minimizing transition time. The gap will decrease as your best possible self becomes more of a reality because you are living in awe-inspiring congruence with your ideals.

True life change happens with a change of habits. The key to cultivating your best self is by developing habits that lift you rather than by focusing on getting rid of "bad" habits. When it comes to identifying which of your current habits are helpful, which are not helpful, and which are neutral or "trick" habits, ask yourself three questions.

3.1. Self-reflection and awareness

Aisha is a really bright and ambitious individual. She thought that the most important thing in her life was doing well at work, and she put all her effort into her career. She knew there was something wrong, and she could not have it until she came across a horrible situation that might spark her awareness. One evening, she felt sick immediately after her 12-hour marathon working, and she realized that she had not eaten since the morning. It was a simple dinner of the day nearby her luxury apartment, and then she fell asleep, so tired that she wet her work clothes with the lights on. Her maid found her unconscious in a dark room, covered with work schedules bellowing from an abandoned cell phone and sheets of worried messages.

On her dinner table, the plate was full of flowerless vegetables. The maid was horrified, but she never uttered a word. When Aisha woke up and was unable to walk due to dehydration, she rushed to the hospital, and the diagnosis was confirmed. Her boss warned her that taking some time off was not ideal due to tight timelines, but of course, Aisha did not listen.

One habit that successful people have mastered is self-reflection and awareness. They have a good understanding of their personality, which allows them to interact with others better. Most importantly, they know their own strengths and weaknesses. It seems like some people come into the world with this innate strength, while we are the unlucky souls that have to work hard to be self-aware. Someday, we stumble upon the wrong place or the wrong friends or find ourselves in the wrong situation because we never spend time learning about ourselves. According to Joseph Foster in his book "Habits Heroes: Building You the Life You Want One Habit At A Time," self-awareness is one of the most important elements of success because it allows us to build habits that cater to our most important needs. Let's look at this scenario.

3.2. Common habits to watch out for

The habit of mediocrity spares us from responsibility. Life is good enough, there is no need for me to strive further. Change is uncomfortable. Failing is my biggest fear. The struggles I'm used to are good enough for me. Habits maintain homeostasis. No need to change. Life is good enough. Just enough is comfortable. Stop. (This is an abrupt stop). The things we fail to do because we are just drifting by in our comfortable life haunt us. "Why didn't I start this earlier?" Better yet, does it display our suffering? How have bad habits hardened our hearts so much that we fail to get up and help? The very thought of that question, to be honest, is bone chilling. The lesson is clear. Don't give in to the siren song of just enough.

Avoid emptiness. Run the full distance. Not having a purpose, true purpose, is draining. Never give into the habit of showing up to leave your mark and legacy on this planet because as we will see - nothing good ever came from just showing up.

Mediocre life. Just getting by. "Bleh" moments. Drowning sorrows every day. Okay, maybe that is a bit dramatic, but the feeling of mediocrity is real. The habit is to show up just to put in your time and protect our ego, or to do things we're used to doing. The habit of cowardice develops from our desire to protect our ego. The sheer pleasure that fixed habits provide blunts our awareness of the present experience. We become lost in a colorful, complex world and never actually appreciate it. We fast forward through days and months without actually living. An empty, mediocre life is a meaningless life.

CHAPTER 4

Creating Positive Habits

Whatever habit you have, the main operative principle at work is activation built-in automaticity. To better see this, consider the three-step process by which a habit is formed, one in which one has gained or mastered a later skill. This is why employees after their first weeks, pharmacy students during training in their pharmacy school, settle on the next logical problem through the therapeutic cascade to follow without a pharmacist having to consciously drag into each stage. Why do toothpaste lovers leave the bathroom to brush their bodies? Because the amygdala quickly pairs with sensory signals. It urges us from our awareness directly into the bathroom. The most surprising finding is that before any conscious awareness of the correspondence between the cue and response emerged, the rats, in essence, acted in anticipation of the AV activation. The rats' connection to compulsive exercise as they pop out of the bed was thinking: Hold a fawn to the lure triggers, go to the gym, done!

"A habit is something you do where you've done it for so long you actually don't even really have to think about what to do next," said Orny Adams on the first season of the NBC series America's Got Talent. "It's actually harder to not do it." Any word that describes who you are (happy, brooding, overweight, active, lazy, persistent, focused, aimless, loving, rude) could be one word, which describes the sum of the countless things you tend to do automatically. All day you are in the process of making or reinforcing habits. The only question is, what sort of habits are you creating? Any habit can be classed as either helpful or toxic. Habits that don't have any evident impact or that one sees as benign tilt in the dangerous direction. The habits you have either frame you for joy or sadness, success or failure, excellence or mediocrity.

4.1. Setting goals for habit change

A long-term commitment to change is most advantageous, but it requires vigilant tracking, accountability to others, and periodic use of compensatory behaviors. Long-term habit change successes are less frequent among individuals who view successful change as having a problem disappear, rather than remain under control, and whose plans depend on being motivated to engage in behavior. Use a values hierarchy with other strategies. Many strategies are available to help you change a health habit. This article advocates using the values hierarchy as a framework to develop not just change strategies (consistent with the remainder of the integrative model), but the long-term learning necessary to sustain pattern changes and the psychological flexibility needed to creatively problem-solve during more stressful environmental challenges.

This is the most straightforward application of a values hierarchy: setting a goal for habit change. As you reflect and develop action steps to help you meet your goal, keep in mind existing time commitments, obligations to others, and the resources available to you. Goals such as finding time for moderate aerobic exercise of 30 minutes, five times a week, doing both strength and flexibility training, or managing your weight over time are most likely to succeed if you have an organized plan based on feedback from others—

particularly those undergoing similar habit change. Keep in mind the sequence of habit change, a process where nearly everyone repeats failed attempts prior to long-term changes. It is unusual to have successful early repetitions of the behavior.

4.2. Strategies for successful habit formation

Charles Duhigg, the author of The Power of Habit (2012), is also an advocate of using commitment contracts to help people stick to their new habits. Commitment contracts are a special type of agreement where you make a deal that you will do something, and if you do not follow through, you will have to pay money. Typically, commitment contracts require you to report on a regular basis to an accountability partner – such as a friend or a charity. All of the data recorded will be evidence that you are sticking to your new habit. For example, you might agree to run three times a week or eat a low-fat, low-sugar diet and if you did not do so and you miss a single workout, you would have to pay $100.00 to a charity you hate, like the American Nazi Party or the Ku Klux Klan. If you had a friend monitor your progress, it would be difficult for you to escape without facing some repercussions. A commitment contract can be a particularly helpful tool, because when people have to put their money where their mouths are on their habit development goals, they are more likely to stick to their goals.

One great strategy to help you adopt a new habit is to find a habit partner who will adopt the same habit with you, and you can support each other as you try to take on your challenge. People who team up with a friend to try to lose weight together are more successful than people who try to lose weight alone, because they can team up to help motivate each other and work together to find solutions to challenges. In one study, people who went on a diet with at least one friend lost more weight than dieters who were assigned to diet without any friends. Having a friend go on a diet with

14 – T.J. RAVENSCROFT

you can be fun, and if your friend also commits to waking up early in the morning to go on a run with you, you are even more likely to stick to your routine because then you are accountable to not only yourself but also to your friend.

4.3. Overcoming obstacles and setbacks

In simplest terms, we need to strengthen the weak points in our approach. That need may be the building of a habit that should have provided immediate support or a coping device but didn't. The individual or caregiver can perform an activity reconnaissance before they engage in the situation that resulted in the setback. This reconnaissance should be reflective in that it begins by recalling specific situations that required a certain set of skills. The next point is to internally or externally set the habits that worked and immediately after, the opposite, i.e. what skills through habits are missing. Lastly, the next step involves integrating the skills before the activities occur.

It's no secret we will encounter setbacks almost as soon as we set out. Just because it's common doesn't mean it has to be discouraging. This is going to be a marathon, not a sprint. For right now, decorating your cube with a rabbit or printing out a picture of the tortoise is a great idea. Along the way, we're faced with a lot of obstacles, setbacks, restraints, or weaknesses that have marginalized us in the past. Returns and we lose our focus. In the means to success, we may encounter learning disabilities, attention deficits, physical limitations, content areas for which we have very little interest, and social situations that take over our lives, i.e. births, deaths, moving, marriage, or the absence of it. These situations do have a reflection in reality for our habits. It is critically important that failures or setbacks are reflected upon. We assess the element(s) of our approach that may have weakened the habit we have been earnestly pursuing.

CHAPTER 5

Breaking Negative Habits

The first secret toward breaking a bad habit is to establish clear goals for the new behavior. "Crisp, specific goals. Blurry goals engender jammed-wrapped habits." Following this advice makes good sense from the principles discussed earlier. Specific goals focus attention. They direct action toward desired outcomes. They affect persistence. Specific goals also help to develop new habits by making it clear how to reach desired outcomes. How could a doctor help a heart attack patient quit smoking if the patient lacked specific goals? After counseling the patient about potential problems of smoking, the doctor's next activity would be to ask the patient to make specific plans to stop. Just asking the patient about those plans would increase the chances the patient would act on them. Interdepartmental politics within organizations can also spring from blurred goals of habit breaking. One department involved in advertisements for a distributor of wooden furniture assured its sales department that working with the distributor was a good idea. This department made no specific plans to do so, ho." Now all managers of Weber's department suppose that the schmiel style of Habits, are poorly functioning fools," she said during a lull. They have failed to outline key steps that can be taken to begin moving the distributor product. They have not specified goals, objectives, and subgoals toion. Serena is a thoughtful person. She generated subgoals based on her Thursday meeting. She had already often made engender selling distributor products. She herself outlined top. However, no one else in the office did more than talk incessantly about meeting scheduled reinforcement goals. As a consequence, salespeople faced high ambiguity, talked about mixed goals, and confronted breeding resentment about interdepartmental politics. The office's inaction if specific command structured the habit-breaking process. The next four Secrets of Habit Breaking provide this structure.

All of us need to break at least one bad habit. We may be comfortable with treating others inappropriately. We use money in a way that is contrary to our long-term financial interests. We find ourselves reacting to personal mistakes or problems by giving up rather than fixing the problem. We drink more alcohol than we should. Habit breaking is one personal change that is pervasive. This chapter gives specific recommendations on how to break a huge variety of bad habits. The scientific literature on habit breaking has its gaps, but the evidence firmly supports the recommendations I make. That's not to say that every one of my recommendations will work for every habit, but the scientific evidence supports using them. Most of them are spread across three broad categories, best done together. These are: setting goals for the new habit; using "The Seven Secrets of Habit Breaking" as a template for other habit-breaking approaches; and using new situations to interrupt old habits. The remaining three are older, more limited strategies.

5.1. Understanding the root causes of negative habits

Remember, there are 86,400 seconds each day. For humans, these seconds can make the greatest change. If guilt doesn't create transformation, you'll make the same mistake again. The job is to be aware when your mind tries to play virtual imagery with you or start framing interpretation about your neighbors based on jealousy. The expectation you create will eventually create a reality for you. The thorough understanding of the expectancy theory is an excellent theory on the power of expectation. Your way of thinking necessitates respect, the way you visualize your expectation based on belief and eventually increase your thinking energy and move everything towards its manifestation. Your habits are created one step at a time. The same thing applies to smooth relapse (sabotage), unlike the first relapse which could sabotage over the years in seconds at its initial stage.

The root of any problem is its intellectual cause, the way we think. The power of your thought influences your habits. Your way of thinking influences everything: your perception, interpretations, and expectations. This is all about RET, Rational Emotive Theory - it states that your belief precedes your behavior. You are the master of your own self; you have your own life's manual and you and only you are capable of driving it. There are a lot of people who think of themselves as "puppets" of someone; as if the entire world were destined to bring them down. These are the people who can focus on negative things like negative media, friends' propaganda, thieves calling someone's destiny, jealousy, influential discouragement folk, and other obstacles, in the process pulling their thinking energy down to nothing.

5.2. Techniques for breaking bad habits

To replace bad habits with good ones, we need to be very aware of our most frequent behaviors, identifying undesirable habits that consume a lot of our time, have a negative impact on our health, or hinder our progress. Self-awareness is the first skill you should develop to break a bad habit. The best way to overcome bad habits is to define a new course of action that is equally capable of bringing the same satisfaction that emerges from them. Find distracting activities to help you overcome your cravings. Keep active and motivated, incentives help. The increase in our productive capacity directly affects our ability to accomplish goals, helps to develop new habits and eliminate others that don't add value to our lives. To do this, have a clear and concise plan: every time you take action oriented towards achieving a goal, record your results, so it is possible to quantify your productivity over time, and check the increase.

So much of success in life is about habits – things we do regularly versus things we do irregularly. Some habits are supportive of the person you're trying to become and "make your life attractive" while others can be like anchors that bind. These can slow you down in critical moments and keep us from realizing our true potential. So, it is crucial to put new habits in place of these negative patterns of behavior that no longer serve you or your greater good. Changing habits isn't propaedeutically easy but it is possible with commitment, discipline and sometimes some ingenuity and creativity. Breaking bad habits can be difficult, but there are many natural, safe, and non-invasive ways to break your bad habits. The following 11 tips will get you on the road to breaking your bad habits and replacing them with good ones.

5.3. Maintaining progress and preventing relapse

You must remember one thing. You are not an addict, you are not a slave to your desires. Every action you take is a conscious one. Your desires do not control you, but you are in control of what you do. Despite failures, despite obstacles – you ultimately decide the outcome of your life. If you want to stay where you are, you do not have to change anything. Your habits will stay the same – no hesitation there. If you truly, genuinely want to change, you are the only one who can make that conscious decision and stick to it.

There is no way to totally prevent relapse while working on maintenance. Just because you haven't smoked a cigarette doesn't mean that one day in the future you might slip and stumble. Relapses do happen. Using the previous flow chart in a modified way, if you notice a significant decline, and you are now three weeks away from your last forum post – you are one day, two days, three days, or however many days away from successfully resetting that habit to commence again.

Maintenance is about making small, incremental changes, reminders, adjustments, repeating successes, and exploring different behavior patterns. The bigger, more important question to be addressed is: how do you preserve and what can one do to prevent a relapse? How to stop slipping into a life of old habits when you are consistent for a couple of months and then, within no time, you are back to square one? The reason maintenance is so difficult is because it is a full-time challenge. It is something that you have to work at every day.

CHAPTER 6

Habit Stacking and Habit Tracking

Resistance during the first few days makes or breaks a new habit. For this, performance tracking is key. It is absolutely required for new habits and very helpful for existing habits. This is the reason pedometers work so well. Very simple, very effective. Recording the habits you have just performed. Many consider it useless as it doesn't help in doing the habit, but it's one of the reasons it works more effectively than compulsive workouts and meditation plans. Writing on a sheet of paper all the tasks to do that day helps enhance productivity because it also makes them automatic. Making the productive task habitual is the second step, but a crucial one, and it all begins with tracking each time it is performed. To track a habit, you must first define its minimum. How shall you measure the habit daily? Once daily, twice daily... or more frequent? Each defined result is a source of focus the next time it's performed. The shadows of the goals you have set for performing the habit often keep you performing it. Tracking is best used with habit stacking in the quest to form new habits and a better life.

The one habit you need for success with all the others is habit stacking. It means choosing an existing habit to be your cue to perform a new habit. The new habit is not something that you have to think about; it is something that happens in sequence after your decision to do it, as you perform an existing habit. Hence, this is also called chaining. A good example of this is using toothpaste as a cue that it's time to do pushups. Or walking to your car as a cue to stop at the mailroom to ask for mail. Habit stacking makes your habits automatic and hence easier to form. Just keep in mind that the habit you shall choose as a cue must be an existing habit, not a new habit, and it should also be one that gets regularly performed. Once you start doing it frequently, it is never forgotten and so the new habit will neither.

6.1. Combining habits for efficiency

Once you have developed the habit of doing 2 push-ups every morning, you can gradually increase the number of push-ups you do to however many you would like using reinforcement of whatever type you like. Once you are consistently doing strength exercises, you can add a new habit like stretching before the strength exercises. Once that feels like a regular part of your day, you might add a new habit like doing moderate exercise outside four or five times a week. This can become a habit you have attached to the end of your workday that feels automatic because your other habits have merged into the giant habit of doing physical activity. It ends up looking something like the following graphics. After you have developed a suite of habits around a particular area of your life, those habits will spontaneously merge into one giant habit that doesn't require motivation, self-control, or a great deal of thinking to enact. You effectively outsource your motivation and self-control to your environment through the development of your habits.

So, how does a habit cascade look in reality? Let us take physical activity as an example. If you are just starting out (or you have never really been very active) and you want to develop a new habit, the most common advice is to begin with a very small step that you will be able to keep consistently. It might be something like: "Do 2 push-ups immediately after waking up." Consistency here is key - the goal isn't just to do 2 push-ups but to develop the habit of doing push-ups every morning.

6.2. Using technology and tools for habit tracking

There's an intuitive step that many people make when they are learning about habit-building tools: to start thinking up how these tools could be used in their personal and professional lives to help them manage time and things in general. I also very much see habit-building improvement as something that could be improved by tracking carefully, through the use of apps or otherwise. But by using technology in these ways, we're often missing an important application of the technology: mindset development and personal growth. By also paying attention to how behaviors affect the way we experience life, we'll speak, we are empowered to take control over it to the extent that we can. Oftentimes, just the act of tracking can help to enlighten, solely because you pay more attention.

But there's a second, less talked about, type of data that can be very powerful when tracked. The by-products of human behavior can be reflections of our inner selves. Tracking tools such as the Quantified Mind or Lift can be powerful tracking and self-analysis tools that can help individuals get clarity on who they are, or at the very least who they want to be. By reflecting on how different habits are related to mood, sleep, energy levels, or even the most minute details like willpower levels (tracking willpower? Sure, using this app), you start to be able to find relationships between habits and how life is being experienced.

Tracking technology has become extremely popular in the personal health and wellness industry. Sales numbers for wearables like the Jawbone and Fitbit are strong and growing every year. There are countless apps available that can track any number of personal biometrics and activities. This type of self-analysis can be an extremely powerful tool in personal development. The old adage, "What gets measured, gets managed" is well understood from a personal level. Being able to measure different habit details like the number of workouts a week, the number of times you eat vegetables, and how many hours a night of sleep can be very powerful in behavior change because it's easy to see where you're improving, what is actually happening compared to what is thought to be happening, and how different habits might be related to one another.

CHAPTER 7

The Power of Habit in Personal Development

Hypothesis: "Has personal development been better characterized as a change brought about only through the formation of new habits?" In response to the Pillar of Achievement question of "What then is personal development?" it is hypothesized that any character exchange will conclude that personal development perhaps better reflects a change that occurs only through the formation of new habits. Every stated positive personal change character following the semantics code is rationally classifiable as a habit. This involved (1) identifying a character as a habit, (2) associating a sequence of characters with an identical habit, and (3) re-establishing this habit if lost. Critics maintaining that habits only account for 99% of the labeled change also concur with the grand hypothesis. This research formally introduces the seven habits of highly personal people. Defined as only being habit-composed humans, it could be proposed that all of these people are highly habit-composed due to the holistic dominance of the character exchange. Furthermore, just as Stephen R. Covey claimed great success by directly treating the habits of readers in his bestseller "The 7 Habits of Highly Effective People," it is theorized that these same seven habits could potentially work for all 'very highly' personal individuals in achieving a recurring type of quantifiable success.

As early as 1786, William Paley rightly surmised this human habit-forming nature: "The chief use of habit, in moral cases, is to produce the effect of compound interest of money, by saving time and increasing vigilance." Exemplifying this human quality, Jesus (c. 4 B.C./A.D. 30) asked, "Which of you, desiring to build a tower, does not first sit down and count the cost, whether he has enough to complete it?" Engagements are monetarily rewarding to the popular self-help industry, which made "millions off of the American public's bottomless appetite for self-improvement" in 2005. Famous authors like Stephen R. Covey's "The 7 Habits of Highly Effective People: Powerful Lessons in Personal Change," habit writer Charles Duhigg wrote, "Why don't we have a habit for saving?" Of the about 650 human engagement topics found in a bookstore chain, about yet habit makes the list. Moreover, today's most subscribed to YouTube channels statistically teach lifestyle habits to most college-age individuals.

7.1. Habits for personal growth and success

Identity is a crucial aspect of personal growth. In the world of business and development, it is understood that individuals don't typically gain advantages by building up on their weaknesses. What really sets them apart is when they develop their strengths. In the same way, spending time sweating over little things sets top performers apart. They focus their energy on strengthening the necessary skills and building relationships that other people ignore. One of the biggest drawbacks to setting ambitious goals is that it can create overwhelming demands. Great leaders don't simply set high goals; they focus on the habits they need to develop in order to reach them. During the journey of personal development, you will experience highs and lows, successes and failures. Sometimes it will seem as though you are going backward but remember, personal development isn't a linear progression.

Have you ever wanted to be someone, but didn't know how? You know you're capable of more than you're doing right now, but you haven't been able to discover exactly what you need to do to reach your full potential. Self-improvement is like a never-ending journey of self-discovery with the lasting effect of success and prosperity. You can almost think of it as an athlete training to enhance their skills, or even an actor honing their craft to be better in their next performance. Read on and apply these habits and principles to become the person you've always wanted to be.

7.2. Cultivating a growth mindset

When you find yourself in this type of pickle, one way forward is to easily, readily and genuinely switch your mindset. It's true that the more you use a particular mindset, the stronger it gets. But it doesn't mean that you can't switch your mindset. So if you are truly committed to living your life as a lifelong learner, then don't you owe it to yourself to at least take the first baby step to try on this new mindset and see what happens? Once you do that first step of trying on a growth mindset, it's good to do your very best to start flexing your growing growth muscles in small, doable steps. At first, it might just be a tiny baby step at a time, but positive change is still positive change. With practice, you will get better at it and also realize that the process of learning feels so much better and is more rewarding than staying stuck.

The most helpful idea when you make a mistake—as we all do— is to remember that making mistakes is just part of the learning process. People who have a growth mindset believe that failures and mistakes allow them to learn and improve, while people who have a fixed mindset believe that their mistakes show that they don't have the ability to succeed. However, even if you generally have a growth mindset, it's still common to have situations when you have a fixed mindset. Most people do. Perhaps you are in this situation right now!

CHAPTER 8

Habit Heroes: Real Life Success Stories

November was the inaugural month of what would eventually become the "Habit Heroes" series. I named it "Habit Masters" and featured the first four months of articles covered under that name. Truly, my personal favorite "Habit Heroes" interview. Jeremy, who has a background in exercise science, was able to achieve one of the most incredible personal transformations I've ever heard of through his "Lifestyle Transformation Program". He is the creator of two popular websites, Fit and Marry and Live More Awesome, and shares a lot of wonderful strategies for improving physical and mental health, as well as personal development at Real Meaningful Life. We talk about Jeremy's favorite habits, his program, and where he's being challenged at the moment in his life. One of the interviews from my first book. Mike, who used to weigh over 300 pounds, educates us on "potential" habits that must be completed first and how to supplement them with mindfulness habits.

In 2013, I had the idea to start a Habit Heroes series on Lifehack. Each month, I would interview someone who had successfully turned their life around and learn silently shared insights. These were the early beginnings of the Habit Heroes series. Six months later, "Building the Life You Want One Habit At a Time" (my first book) was produced from those interviews. These are all of the amazing success stories that started it all:

8.1. Inspiring stories of habit transformation

After a year of anthropological participant observation, Robinson documented 110 habits handwritten on a sheet of exercise paper. The most impressive aspect of the habits, which would result in chronic illness and disease reversal, came from the respondents' ages. "99%" of them were over the age of 74. Robinson was confounded by the observation until Wisdom appeared in the middle of the night in a dream to ask if she had finished the documentation. Then Wisdom said, "If you are as smart as everyone believes you are, and you have no bias for any way of life but your primary allegiance is to improve your people's quality of life, copy the elderly." With five words, Wisdom summarized the primary discovery of chronic illness: the elderly in the community lived about seven (7) decades of their lives before developing chronic conditions. I choose to refer to the beginning of this discovery as the creation of a lifestyle blueprint. This idea disputes the approach of failures springs from the founders of the lifestyle-related practices worldwide.

Health educator and coach, Gain Robinson, became captivated by the possibility of habit transformation after attending a medical conference on chronic illness in the United States in 1992. The speakers presented Ghana, the country of Robinson's birth, as an island of health where chronic illnesses were rare. To help understand how Nigerians could have the same healthy benefits, despite wrestling with similar economic adversity, the 82-year-old family patriarch asked Robinson to spend a year documenting the community's habits.

30 — T.J. RAVENSCROFT

8.2. Lessons learned from Habit Heroes

When the hobby is enjoyment, the probability goes up further. Further, the research I mentioned earlier repeatedly shows similar results – 90% of successful weight loss maintainers used incentives at least some of the time. And the gym membership study reveals that incentivizing gym attendance increases it up to 431%. Habit Heroes is the method of incorporating reward-driven change into weight loss in an organized manner. Habit Heroes encourages others to award stars to only those they care about, showing others what is important, and maximizing the meaning and strength of the reward. Given that we are creatures of habit evidenced by a tendency to eat the same foods every day, for example, to minimize negative habits, we should do the opposite and strive to make sustainable positive habits easy to form, with the use of rewards especially when we're first learning.

Chapter seven not only summarized the lessons I learned from my weight loss journey, it summarized the lessons anyone who is successful in weight loss learns. The first lesson learned: Shift from punishment-based rewards to incentive-based rewards. The habits that lead to weight gain are often deeply ingrained and difficult to change using conventional methods. The second lesson learned: Punishment is a highly ineffective way of creating sustainable change. A method I had been trying to enforce leading up to this weight loss journey that had resulted in mostly failure. The third lesson learned: Rewards can drive change more effectively than punishment. Rewarding myself for going to the gym, for example, led to a much higher probability I would actually go to the gym. Using drawing at the gym as an example, the probability went from 0%, increasing over 400% to a 70% probability.

Milton Keynes UK
Ingram Content Group UK Ltd.
UKHW031400011224
451790UK00009B/130